The Best Practice Is The Lowest Effective Dose
Your Third Psychiatric Consultation

Copyright Applied for 11/03/2019,
All rights reserved, William R. Yee M.D., J.D.

In most cases the best practice is the lowest effective dose of medications. When higher doses are used there must be a significant and substantial justification for using more than the lowest effective dose.

Massive doses of antibiotics for rapid resolution of a fulminant (rapidly progressive) infection in an immune compromised patient is an example of a reasonable exception.

Massive doses are rarely justified because of the risks of respiratory arrest, cardiac arrest, liver failure and renal failure resulting in death. Death trumps any putative benefit of convenience or cost that massive doses of psychotropic medications might reap for the hospital, prison or nursing home.

The patient, family, medical student, law student, MBA in hospital administration and other stake holders need to know why the lowest effective dose is the best practice.

The first principle that the stakeholders should understand is the notion of physiologic reserves.

Physiologic reserves are the excess liver capacity, the excess renal capacity, the excess buffering for exposure to acids or bases, the excess tolerance to heat or cold, the excess tolerance to carbon monoxide, the excess capacity to tolerate atropine, or QT prolonging drugs before there is permanent injury or death. Other parameters are easily found by looking at the list of side effects in the FDA Prescription Drug Labeling. This includes the prescribing information, package insert, professional labeling, direction circular and package circular.

I suggest the reader log on to the internet and find the package insert, the professional labeling, the direction circular and the package circular for any medication that they, their family and friends take.

Before the patient takes the first pill he should read and understand the package insert that is given by the pharmacy with the medication.

My exposure to psychotropic medications began in Lafayette Clinic, in Detroit Michigan in 1972.

Lafayette Clinic was a psychiatric hospital operated by the Michigan Department of Mental Health.

At one time there were sixteen state psychiatric hospitals in Michigan.

At this time there are only three state psychiatric hospitals in Michigan:

1. Caro Center, in Caro, Michigan
2. Kalamazoo Psychiatric Center, in Kalamazoo, Michigan and
3. Walter Reuther Psychiatric Hospital, in Westland, Michigan

Lafayette Clinic was unique among the state operated hospitals in Michigan. It was a research hospital under the direction of Dr. Jacques Gottlieb.

All the patients admitted to Lafayette Clinic had to sign consent to be part of experimental research that could be published.

I was told that one research project involved ten to fifteen grams of Thorazine a day.

I don't know if this was a mistake on the speaker's part, or merely an attempt to deceive a new and naïve resident in psychiatric training. I merely repeat the statement to give the reader a flavor of the environment I was training under in nineteen seventy-two.

I do know that one to three thousand milligrams a day of Thorazine was within the range of possibilities at that time.

A patient at Lafayette Clinic died from hypothermia caused by Thorazine. After that death, patients were monitored daily for blood pressure, pulse, temperature, and somatic complaints.
Current guidelines for Thorazine allow up to two thousand milligrams of Thorazine a day for mania and schizophrenic psychosis.

When I was at Northville State Hospital from 1973 to 1975, I gave a floridly psychotic patient one hundred milligrams of Thorazine, and he slept for three days. He asked me to reduce the dose, so I changed the dose of Thorazine from one hundred milligrams at bedtime to fifty milligrams at bedtime. He did well after the medication reduction was ordered.

In that case I do not know if the patient was manic or schizophrenic and responded to the one hundred milligrams of Thorazine. He may have been psychotic from methamphetamine and when he stopped taking the methamphetamine, he may have slept for three days as part of his withdrawal from methamphetamine rather than a side effect of the Thorazine. In either case, a psychotic episode is often broken by a period of sound sleep.

In psychotic states it is better to induce sleep with Thorazine than with a sleeping pill like Ambien which has psychotic and behavioral side effects

Since that time, I have always favored low dose psychotropic medications for two reasons.
1. First, I did not see much improvement with medication increases after the initial dose.
2. Second, I saw severe side effects with medication increases after the first dose.

There are literally hundreds of side effects for any medication. Each side effect is a part of the physiologic reserve that has been stressed past its normal capacity to compensate back to the baseline optimum physiologic function.

A perceived side effect is an indication that the physiologic reserve is being stressed past the body's normal ability to maintain the optimum homeostatic balance.

The most significant physiologic reserves are listed under the Black Box Warnings in the package insert. Black Box Warnings usually identify sudden death as a side effect.

The next most significant physiologic reserves are listed under the side effects of an overdose of a medication.

The least urgent side effects are then listed as common side effects and rare side effects. Occasionally, rare side effects can be very urgent. In the vulnerable patient a common side effect can be urgent. Vulnerable patients are the very young, the very old and the very sick.

Stress on the physiologic reserve can be acute with immediate adverse effect such as allergic reactions or death.

Stress on physiologic reserves can be chronic with delayed effects such as weight gain, diabetes, kidney failure, and liver failure.

Tardive dyskinesia and enlarged breasts with milk production in males due to prolactin elevation are relatively common delayed side effects with antipsychotic medications.

When I was at Northville State Hospital
The literature indicated that after a year or two in a state hospital about fifty percent of the patients had tardive dyskinesia. This was because in state hospitals the practice was to prescribe very high doses of antipsychotic medications. Drug free holidays were common.

The best example of an acute stress on physiologic reserve is the LD50. The physiologic reserves are quickly overwhelmed with masses doses of water and other substances.
The LD50 is the dose at which half the population dies when taken rapidly.

Just about everything has an LD50. The LD50 for water is Six liters. Half the people who drink six liters of water rapidly die from water intoxication.

The LD50 for medications is not known precisely as it is not ethical to experiment on humans to find out what the LD50 of medications are.

Aspirin is a good example. The exact LD50 for aspirin is not known. However, review of large number of overdoses results in a consensus that 150 mg/kg or 6.5 g of aspirin is a lethal dose. For a 100kg man, (220 pounds), a lethal dose is between 6.5 and 15 grams of aspirin.

Fifteen grams of aspirin are equal to forty-six, (46), 325 milligram aspirin tablets or one hundred and eighty-five, (185) 81 milligram tablets.

You can buy a thousand 325 milligram tablets for ten dollars online.

The LD50 for amitriptyline is not known. The maximum daily dose of amitriptyline is 300mg a night for the treatment of depression,

I read an anecdotal report of a patient dying after taking 1500mg, a five-day supply of amitriptyline.

Historically, amitriptyline is the most common cause of death by overdose among the antidepressants accounting for about one third of those deaths. This is because tricyclic antidepressants tend to be the most toxic as compared to other psychotropic medications.

Symptoms of amitriptyline overdose prior to death include hypothermia, respiratory depression and arrest, coma, seizures, abnormal tendon reflexes, confusion, agitation, myoclonic jerks, excessively brisk reflexes and extensor (upgoing) plantar reflexes, cardiac arrhythmias, bundle branch block, cardiac arrest, low blood pressure, circulatory collapse, dilated pupils, blurred vision, tachycardia, vasodilation, urinary retention, decreased gastrointestinal motility, decreased bronchial secretions, dry mucous membranes, hot dry skin, tachycardia.

Many of these amitriptyline side effects are atropine side effects shared with many other medications on the Beers List of medications.

In the real world, overdose is usually in combination with benzodiazepines, alcohol and other substances that increase the risk of respiratory arrest and death.

Karen Ann Quinlan (March 29, 1954 – June 11, 1985) is a famous example of drug overdose by multiple agents.

Opiates often result in death from respiratory arrest when combined with benzodiazepines, sleeping pills, and alcohol.

Any medication side effect is toxicity that could lead to injury or death in the near term or the far term depending upon the patient's DNA and other intervening variables including diet, other medications, stress from heat or cold, etc.

Look up the symptoms of overdose to understand the toxicity of your medications. After Elavil toxicity of other psychotropic medications starting with the most toxic to the least toxic follows:
1. monoamine oxidase inhibitor with cheese
2. tricyclic antidepressants

3. Lithium with a narrow therapeutic window. Excessive heat or exercise can result in toxicity and death with lithium.
4. venlafaxine
5. valproic acid
6. bupropion
7. quetiapine
8. olanzapine
9. ziprasidone
10. carbamazepine
11. Desvenlafaxine.

Many psychotropic medications are omitted from the above list because toxicity in terms of LD50 and death is really not known very well.

The reason that the LD50 is not known is because most overdoses are with a mixture of medications, alcohol, and street drugs. Listing the relative toxicity has very limited value as a result.

Chronic exposure to psychotropic medications can result in death from liver failure, kidney failure, pancreatitis, loss of white cells, loss of red calls, weight gain, diabetes, hypertension, stroke, low sodium, etc.

Other long, term side effects include polycystic ovaries from Depakote and tardive dyskinesia from antipsychotic and other medications.

Tardive dyskinesia is not a trivial matter. It is abnormal motor movements at rest. It is cosmetically disfiguring, and patients have committed suicide on that basis. The end stage of tardive dyskinesia results in difficulty in breathing and swallowing. When severe, the patient has to have a gastrotomy for a feeding tube directly to the stomach and a tracheotomy for breathing to bypass the mouth, nose, and throat compromised by a movement disorder.

It would require hours of education with questions to ascertain adequate understanding of the hundreds of side effects of each medication.

I generally advise the patient to read the package insert, and if the patient does not understand something or is concerned, the patient can defer taking the medication until after making additional appointments to review the package insert before starting the medication.

The patient and family should understand the trajectory of physiologic reserves from birth to death. Generally physiologic reserves are limited at birth and increase with maturation. Senescent deterioration in late life results in loss of physiologic reserves and eventual placement into an Alzheimer's Unit of a nursing home.

At birth the baby does not sleep through the night. The baby generally sleeps through the night at four to sixth months, acquires teeth in the first year, learns to walk at about one, learns to talk at about one and is potty trained by the age of two or three.

In later years, senescent changes tend to mirror the maturation of the baby.

In the last decade of life people tend to lose their teeth. They tend to lose, bowel and bladder control, the ability to sleep through the night, social sensibilities, and modesty. Not closing the bathroom door, not zipping up, not dressing with modesty, irritability, rudeness, coarsening of language and behaviors can all be signs of senescent deterioration and dementia.

The loss of frontal lobe executive functions is the basis of most of the deterioration requiring placement in a secure Alzheimer's Unit.

The limited physiologic reserves and the ethics of medical experimentation on children combine to limit the number of medications that are FDA approves for children.

The off-label use of psychotropic medications for children is very common, and is an example of experimentation without the benefits of FDA ethics committees and other safeguards.

Medications are avoided in infants and tapered with senescent deterioration in late life.

The best practice is the lowest effective dose of medication at any age.
The practice of the lowest effective dose is reflected in the Beers Criteria. Look up Geriatric Society Beers Criteria for Potentially Inappropriate Medication Use in Older Adults.

Physiologic age is not the same as calendar age. The physician, family, and patient need to be aware of the fact that each individual enters senescent decline at a different time and rate.

Also, loss of physiologic reserves can by masked by a robust physical appearance.

Medications are usually not cures for mental illnesses. They usually are treatments with some benefit and some side effects and on average only reduce symptoms by twenty to thirty percent.

The patient passes judgment on whether the benefit justifies the time, cost, and side effects. He does this by taking the medication or not taking the medication.

Insulin is such a good treatment for diabetes that it would be considered malpractice to routinely recommend against the use of insulin for all patients with diabetes. No psychotropic medication has reached this status for the treatment of mental illness.

Thirty percent of depressed patients do not respond to antidepressant medications.

Thirty percent of schizophrenic patients do not respond to antipsychotic medications.

Forty percent of patients with obsessive compulsive disorder do not respond to medications for obsessive compulsive disorder.

Fifty percent of patients do not take the medications prescribed by doctors.

The pharmaceutical industry is well known for false advertising resulting in lawsuits and hundreds of millions of dollars in penalties and fines.

The reader should go on to the internet and read about **Pfizer paying $325** million plus $430 million for a total of $945 million for advertising the benefits of gabapentin/Neurontin for bipolar disorder, ADHD, migraine headaches and other types of pain.

In general, the pharmaceutical industry promotes the use of psychotropic medications in a manner that brings patients to my office with expectations of cures as opposed to limited realistic expectations of modest improvements in symptoms.

Much of the research on medications is funded by the pharmaceutical industry. Unfavorable research is often filed away and not published.

As a result, physicians have a skewed view of the medications advertised and sold. The risk benefit balance is misrepresented with more benefit and less risk than actually exist. Seldane, and many other medications have been taken off the market in many countries because of severe and unexpected side effects not reported in early studies that resulted in a license to sell the medications.

I began prescribing psychotropic medications in 1972 at Lafayette Clinic in Detroit, Michigan.

Patients did not come to me for a treatment of their mental illness. Patients came to me for a cure of their mental illness.

Patients were disappointed with the notion that antidepressant medications could take six to eight weeks to become effective.

I was trained in psychoanalysis, transactional analysis, and other therapies.
I would supplement the medications with psychotherapies. I often continued the psychotherapy without medications.

Many patients were not willing to spend money on medications that only provided a marginal relief from their depression, anxiety, or hallucinations.

The literature reports "noncompliance," at the rate of fifty percent.

I suppose, "noncompliance," is out of line with the principle of, "unconditional positive regard," promoted by the Rogerian School of Psychoanalysis.
"Noncompliance," implies a failure on the patient's part and dismisses a failure on the medication's part or the psychiatrist's part.

I admit that when a medication does not work, I am disappointed in the medication and wish that I had not prescribed it. Does that mean there is something wrong with me?

With Prozac there was a big relief because it was harder to commit suicide with Prozac as compared to Elavil/Amitriptyline.
Prozac was not much better than Elavil for the treatment of depression. Many patients did not like the side effects and refused to take it.

Impotence and loss of sexual drive? Many patients consider medications worse than the mental illness?

There was heavy marketing of Wellbutrin, Seroquel, Effexor, Zyprexa, Clozaril and every psychotropic medication as each medication entered the marketplace. In every case the patient arrived in my office expecting more than what they got. They expected cures and received treatments.

Patients came to my office with high expectations, and eventually were disappointed that there was no substantial improvement, and each medication had a set of unacceptable side effects.

They continued to refuse to take all of the psychotropic medications at the rate of fifty percent or better,

Not only did the patients have disappointment in the medication, but they also had disappointment in me for prescribing the medications. I continued to offer a combination of medications and psychotherapy or psychotherapy without the medications.

"Noncompliance," might be regarded as disrespectful of the consensus among psychiatric patients that psychotropic medications are disappointments.

Why should the pharmaceutical industry expect patients to put up with the high cost of psychotropic medications when the medications have so many side effects and are not cures?

Why should the medical community consider the refusal of medications as, "noncompliance," rather than a vote of no confidence in the medications and notice to the medical community that more is expected, and more is deserved?

The current culture in the pharmaceutical industry and the medical industry should be examined through the lens of a cult.
A cult is characterized by secrecy and control from the top imposed by the members at the bottom. Not all the information known to the cult leaders is shared with the general membership.
The pharmaceutical industry does not share all of the research that it funds.

The pharmaceutical industry misrepresents the benefits and risks. The pharmaceutical industry recruits physicians to misrepresent the risks and benefits of medications. This was done with Neurontin, aka Gabapentin, and many other medications. The pharmaceutical industry has been successful in turning medicine into a cult.

What are other aspects of a cult. The practice of anonymous complaints followed by excommunication or blacklisting is another characteristic of a cult.

I have observed this behavior in state hospitals and prisons.
There is a misperception in state hospitals and prisons that massive doses of medications are necessary for treatment.

Psychiatrists who do not prescribe massive doses of medications or taper medications are subjected to anonymous complaints. The complaints are so anonymous that the people making the complaints are kept secret. The complaint is also kept a secret because it might reveal the person making the complaint.

The psychiatrist is then faced with review by the Peer Review Committee which could lead to loss of hospital privileges, which could prevent accreditation by hospitals and clinics that might offer future employment. It could also lead to denial of malpractice insurance and all possibility of future employment. This is a cult in my book.

Others may have a different opinion.

Consider this thought, among patients who continue taking antipsychotic medications there is a seventeen percent recovery after seven years.

Patients who stop antipsychotic medications have a forty percent recovery after seven years. Why is the fact that patients who stop antipsychotic medications have more than twice the functional recovery after seven years as compared to patients who continue medications not more widely known?

I suppose that it does not serve the pharmaceutical industry to publicize this fact.

I suppose if psychiatric offices are treated as a

business with the revenue stream a priority over patient welfare, it is not a good idea to publicize the fact that patients who stop antipsychotic medications do twice as well as patients who continue their antipsychotic medications.

I suggest that the reader log on to the internet and read the, "Post by Former NIMH Director Thomas Insel: Antipsychotics: Taking the Long View by **Thomas Insel on August 28, 2013.**"

This information has been present since 2013 and has not been given wide consideration as far as I know.

We should give more respect to patients who decide not to take medications.

"Noncompliance," is a vote of no confidence.

Let's look at the number needed to treat, (NNT), for one patient to get better. These numbers are hard to find for psychotropic medications so I will use statins as an example.

Sixty people have to take statins for five years to prevent one heart attack.
Two hundred and sixty people have to take

statins for five years to prevent one stroke. The annual cost of statins is $600 to $1,000 per subject. In addition to the cost of the medication is the cost of the lab tests and office visits. During those five years patients suffer from muscle pain, fatigue, weakness, and rhabdomyolysis which can result in kidney failure.

Log on to the internet and read:

"What are the odds that your medication will help you get better?" by SHARON BEGLEY @sxbegle, JUNE 15, 2016 © 2019 STAT

The number needed to harm, (NNH), is even more difficult to find.

However, read the FDA Prescription Drug Labeling. It will list side effects and percentages of patients with each side effect. That is a good proxy for the number needed to harm, or (NNH).

Let's look at the CATIE trials to grasp the reasonable expectations for benefitting from antipsychotic medications. This trial compared eighteen months of treatment of perphenazine against eighteen months of olanzapine,

quetiapine, risperidone, or ziprasidone.
Only about 25% of subjects in the CATIE trial completed the 18-month trial on the medicine to which they were assigned. That indicates that in general psychotropic medications are not very effective. The dropout rate is rounded to the nearest 5% as follows:

1. 65% olanzapine
2. 75% perphenazine
3. 80% quetiapine
4. 75% risperidone
5. 80% ziprasidone

From the point of view of the patient and the physician there is no meaningful difference in benefit among these medications. Their usefulness is a disappointment with substantial burdens.

Clozapine is the gold standard for the treatment of schizophrenia because of a putative additional benefit with better improvement of social function.

Let us look at the research that allowed Clozapine to be marketed for the treatment of schizophrenia.

Examination of the Clozaril FDA Label reveals black box warnings for Severe Neutropenia, Orthostatic Hypotension, Bradycardia, Syncope (loss of consciousness resulting in falls and injuries), Seizures, Myocarditis, Cardiomyopathy, Mitral Valve Incompetence, and increased mortality in the elderly with dementia.

The reader should be advised that the warning advises of increased death in the elderly with dementia. This is the narrowest interpretation of the research. The research was on the elderly with dementia and not on the elderly with and without dementia. There is no rational basis to think that the elderly without dementia with exposure to Clozaril are safe.

Risk management and common sense would dictate that the above warning should be written in broader terms. The elderly are at increased risk of mortality with the possibility that further research will reveal that the elderly without dementia may not be at increased risk of death.

Further examination of the FDA labeling reveals that the medication was released based upon a mere six, week trial comparing Clozaril to Thorazine aka chlorpromazine.

The measure used was a twenty percent (20%) reduction of symptoms. Twenty percent was considered a clinically significant improvement.

Forty percent of the Clozaril patients had a twenty percent reduction in symptoms after six weeks.

That means that sixty percent of the patients treated with Clozaril did not achieve a clinically significant twenty percent reduction of symptoms.

This compares to four percent of the chlorpromazine patients achieving a twenty percent reduction of symptoms.

A twenty percent reduction in symptoms leaves eighty percent of the symptoms for the patients and the family to deal with.

In a 104 week study, comparing Clozaril to Olanzapine there was a 24% recurrence of suicide attempt or suicidal episodes for Clozaril compared to a 32% rate of recurrence of suicide attempt or suicidal episode for Olanzapine.

The difference was six percent (6%) less suicidal episodes for Clozaril as compared to Olanzapine.

The absolute risk reduction is 32% over two years, You would have to treat three people for two years to reduce suicidal episodes by one.

For Zyprexa you would have to treat four people for two years to reduce suicide episodes by one.

In the case of depression and suicidal episodes, clozapine is clearly indicated if the patient is willing to accept the risk of side effects.

The medical literature in general supports Clozaril as superior to all other antipsychotics and therefore Clozaril is the gold standard for treating schizophrenia.

Clozaril is touted as the antipsychotic that improves social functioning in addition to suppressing hallucinations delusions and paranoia.

However, Meta Analysis of the medical literature, including Cochrane Reviews, reveals many flaws in medical research. Among those flaws are publication bias, short duration studies, and poor quality in data collection,

Recent literature reviews have found that Clozaril does not improve social function.

See, "Clozapine and Psychosocial Function in Schizophrenia: A Systematic Review and Meta-Analysis," Olagunju AT, Clark SR, Baune BT; CNS Drugs. 2018 Nov;32(11):1011-1023. doi: 10.1007/s40263-018-0565-x.

There are reviews that reveal that Clozaril aka Clozapine is not superior to other antipsychotics.

See, "Efficacy, Acceptability, and Tolerability of Antipsychotics in Treatment-Resistant SchizophreniaA Network Meta-analysis," Myrto T. Samara, MD; Markus Dold, MD; Myrsini Gianatsi, MSc; Adriani Nikolakopoulou, MSc; Bartosz Helfer, MSc; Georgia Salanti, PhD; Stefan Leucht,MD

There are articles that indicate that Clozaril is superior to other antipsychotics, but only 40% achieve a benefit and augmentation with aripiprazole, fluoxetine and sodium valproate may provide additional benefit.

See, "Augmentation strategies for clozapine refractory schizophrenia: A systematic review and meta-analysis," Dan J Siskind, Michael Lee, Arul Ravindran, et al, May 6, 2018 Review Article Australian and New Zealand Journal of Psychiatry, https://doi.org/10.1177/0004867418772351

Now let us look at the medical literature for medications used to treat depression.

In general medications used for depression also improve anxiety and panic attacks.

Review of the literature reveals serious weaknesses in the research and there is a strong possibility that there is only a small benefit as compared to placebo and the benefits are inflated.

See, "Considering the methodological limitations in the evidence base of antidepressants for depression: a reanalysis of a network meta-analysis,"
Klaus Munkholm, Asger Sand Paludan-Müller, and Kim Boesen
BMJ Open. 2019; 9(6): e024886.
Published online 2019 Jun 27. doi: 10.1136/bmjopen-2018-024886
PMCID: PMC6597641 PMID: 31248914

Another review reveals only a modest benefit of antidepressant medications.

If 100 is complete relief the medication effect is 30 with seventy percent of symptoms remaining after mediation treatment.

See, "Efficacy and Acceptability of Antidepressants in Acute Depression – What Does the Largest Ever Research Study on Antidepressants Tell Us?
Posted on: March 23, 2018
Last Updated: March 31, 2018
https://psychscenehub.com/psychinsights/efficacy-acceptability-antidepressants-network-meta-analysis/

The placebo effect is equal to 75% of the antidepressant medication effect. That means a sugar pill without medication is 75% as effective as medications prescribed for depression.

See, "Antidepressants and the Placebo Effect," Irving Kirsch, 2008
Z Psychol. 2014; 222(3): 128–134.
doi: 10.1027/2151-2604/a000176
PMCID: PMC4172306
PMID: 25279271

In fact, most of the benefits of medications for the treatment of anxiety and depression is placebo effect and not medication effect.

See, "Placebo Effect in the Treatment of Depression and Anxiety
Front. Psychiatry, 13 June 2019 | https://doi.org/10.3389/fpsyt.2019.00407
Irving Kirsch
Harvard Medical School, Boston, MA, United States

Placebos have no medication and no significant physiologic side effects. Placebos have substantial psychological effects including relief from pain, anxiety, depression, and other symptoms. The idea that there is treatment and the expectation of getting better overcomes the idea that there is mental illness and the need for treatment.

Regardless of the psychotropic or the mental illness, after the failure of the first trial, it is necessary to increase the number of patients treated with each medication increase or medication change for one patient get better,

Less medication and
more psychotherapy,
more meditation,
more physical exercise,
more healthy eating,
more learning,
more social engagement,
more charity,
more fellowship of mankind.
more treating others the way you want to be treated

       Thank you,
            William R. Yee M.D, J.D.

Diet, Exercise, and Sleep Trump Medications
Medication is the Last Option
Your Fourth Psychiatric Consultation

Copyright Applied for 12/15/2019
all rights reserved.
William R. Yee M.D., J.D.

Healthy living habits start in childhood.

"Moderation in All Things," along with the, "Golden Rule," treat others the way you wish to be treated are thoughts that permeate religions, philosophy, and science.

Moderation promotes physical, intellectual and emotional health which make for more effective social, academic, and recreational efforts.

A life of moderation will do more for your physical and mental health than all the pills I can prescribe for you during your lifetime.

The bell-shaped curve describes moderation and extremes in physiologic functions.

One standard deviation encompasses 68% of the population. Two standard deviations encompass 95% of the population.

How does one use standard deviations to describe moderation?

The Bell-Shaped Curve describes distribution of an attribute among the general population.

The notion of moderation must be individualized. Moderation may be described as the zone of maximum value such as optimum blood pressure, optimum quality of life, or longest life span.

Stimulation is one of the most critical variables that is addressed by psychiatrists.

Stimulation is measured along a continuum of low to high stimulation.

Low stimulation is experienced as boredom. Increase the stimulation and you experience pleasure. Increase the stimulation further and you experience stress.

The figure below is a rough example of what a Bell Shape Curve looks like with one standard deviation above and below the average enclosing 68% of the population and two standard deviations above and below the mean enclosing 95% of the population.

There is an optimum amount of stimulation for physical and mental health.

That optimum is different for each individual.

Each individual should explore the boundaries of stimulation to determine what is boring, what is pleasure and what is painful.

The figure below describes insufficient stimulation as boring and too much stimulation as panic.

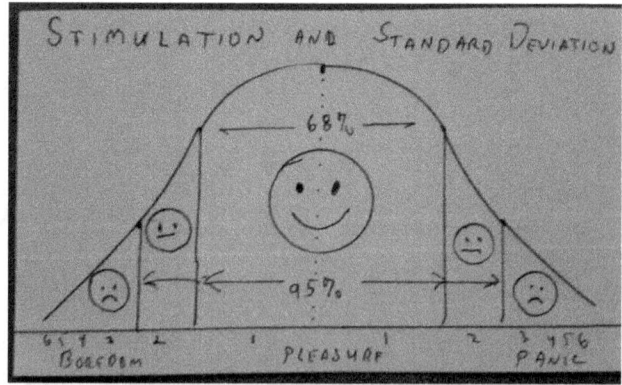

Some people experience excess stimulation as a thrill instead of as a panic. They seek thrills.

It is a matter of point of view and attitude.

Some experience low levels of stimulation as peacefulness instead of boredom.

It is a matter of point of view and attitude.

Attitude determines whether a thrill or panic is experienced. Panic, rage and thrill are all the product of high levels of adrenalin which increases blood pressure and heart rate which is experienced as panic, thrill, or rage.

This book focuses on exercise, sleep, and diet to maximize quality of life.

There are many other activities. As you engage in those activities, you should explore the boundaries of those activities. You should determine how extensive and intensive these activities should be to extract your optimum quality of life.

Let us start with diet.
The first concept that should be considered is the LD50. The LD50 is the lethal dose which kills half of those exposed to that dose.

Consider water. The LD50 for water is six liters. Half of the adults who drink six liters of water rapidly will die.

Consider alcohol. Half of the people who rapidly drink thirteen shots of liquor will die. A shot is 45 milliliters of 40% by volume alcohol.

A teaspoon of caffeine has 3.2 grams of caffeine. About 10 grams or three teaspoons of pure caffeine is a lethal dose.

A moderate or optimal level of water for daily consumption is between eight and fifteen, eight-ounce cups of water for the average adult male and eight to eleven, eight-ounce cups of water for an adult female.

Two to four cups of coffee daily reduce depression and with a reduction of depression one would expect a reduction in suicide. For the average person 70 to 500 milligrams of coffee in the morning reduces the risk of depression and suicide. One cup has 70–140 mg of caffeine.

I rely on: "Coffee, Caffeine, and Risk of Depression Among Women," Michel Lucas, PhD, RD; Fariba Mirzaei, MD, MPH, ScD; An Pan, PhD;

Olivia I. Okereke, MD, SM; Walter C. Willett, MD, DrPH; Éilis J. O'Reilly, ScD; Karestan Koenen, PhD; Alberto Ascherio, MD, DrPH; Arch Intern Med. 2011;171(17):1571-1578. doi:10.1001/archinternmed.2011.393

Fasting is a common practice for religious and other reasons.

There is some evidence that fasting can improve metabolic health and may facilitate weight loss. The issue of fasting merits more research.

Fasting in moderation, like exercise in moderation, is likely to improve quality of life and health.

"Intermittent Fasting and Human Metabolic Health."

Ruth E. Patterson, PhD,1,2 Gail A. Laughlin, PhD,1,2 Dorothy D. Sears, PhD,1,3 Andrea Z. LaCroix, PhD,1,2 Catherine Marinac, BA,1,4 Linda C. Gallo, PhD,5 Sheri J. Hartman, PhD,1,2 Loki Natarajan, PhD,1,2 Carolyn M. Senger, MD,1,2 María Elena Martínez, PhD,1,2 and Adriana Villaseñor, PhD1,2
J Acad Nutr Diet. Author manuscript; available in PMC 2016 Aug 1.

Published in final edited form as:
J Acad Nutr Diet. 2015 Aug; 115(8): 1203–1212.
Published online 2015 Apr 6.
doi: 10.1016/j.jand.2015.02.018
PMCID: PMC4516560
NIHMSID: NIHMS663671
PMID: 25857868

"Coffee and caffeine consumption and depression: A meta-analysis of observational studies."
Wang L, Shen X, Wu Y, Zhang D.
Aust N Z J Psychiatry. 2016 Mar;50(3):228-42. doi: 10.1177/0004867415603131. Epub 2015 Sep 2.

Maintaining healthy eating with a body mass index between 19 and 25 will lengthen life and reduce the risk of health problems.

A healthy BMI for men and women is between 19 and 25. Consult with your doctor.
Approximate healthy weights for BMI of 19-25
Height --- Weight
4'10" ----- 91 to 115 pounds
4'11" ----- 94 to 119 pounds
5'00" ----- 97 to 123 pounds
5'01" ----- 100 to 127 pounds

5'02" ----- 104 to 131 pounds
5'03" ----- 107 to 135 pounds
5'04" ----- 110 to 140 pounds
5'05" ----- 114 to 144 pounds
5'06" ----- 118 to 148 pounds
5'07" ----- 121 to 153 pounds
5'08" ----- 125 to 158 pounds
5'09" ----- 128 to 162 pounds
5'10" ----- 132 to 167 pounds
5'11" ----- 136 to 172 pounds
6'00" ----- 140 to 177 pounds
6'01" ----- 144 to 182 pounds
6'02" ----- 148 to 186 pounds
6'03" ----- 152 to 192 pounds
6'04" ----- 156 to 205 pounds
6'05" ----- 162 to 211 pounds
6'06" ----- 164 to 216 pounds
6'07" ----- 169 to 222 pounds
6'08" ----- 173 to 228 pounds
6'09" ----- 177 to 233 pounds
6'10" ----- 182 to 239 pounds

Let us start with the adverse effects of obesity.

As the BMI rises from 25 to 50 many health problems emerge. The health problems of obesity defeat medications and surgical treatments for obesity.

Obesity increases fat in the belly, liver, heart, brain, prostate gland, arteries, skin and other organs,

Let's start with the brain. Fat in the brain causes the brain to expand. Unfortunately, the brain is in the skull which protects the brain from damage due to blunt trauma such as falls.

When the brain expands it puts pressure on the brain stem and optic nerves which are near openings that relieve pressure on the brain.

The result on the optic nerve is pseudo tumor cerebri. The fat puts pressure on the optic nerve and acts like a false tumor.

Intracranial hypertension from obesity has been reported commonly and can even affect children and adolescents.

Headaches with obesity are a warning sign of intracranial hypertension and pseudotumor cerebri.

When the doctor looks into the eye at the optic nerve, he sees that pseudotumor cerebri causes swelling of the optic nerve which can lead to loss of vision.

Pseudotumor cerebri headaches sometimes manifests as pain behind the eyes.

Sometimes the patient can hear the blood pulsing in the arteries of the head with pseudotumor cerebri.

Intracranial pressure can result in nausea and vomiting that can also occur with subdural hematomas from head injuries.

There may be loss of visual acuity, (loss of the ability to perceive fine details), or loss of portions of the visual fields with pseudotumor cerebri. The most common visual field defect is increase in the blind spot size. The second most common visual defect is loss of portions of the medial or nasal sides of the visual fields in both eyes. The loss of visual acuity and visual fields is associated with chronic papilledema, or chronic swelling of the optic nerve.

Simply said, the longer the patient has swelling of the brain and swelling of the optic nerve, the more likely there will be permanent loss of visual fields and visual acuity.

Respiratory problems are common with obesity and increase in severity with increased obesity.

Accumulation of fat in the chest and abdomen results in mechanical compression of the diaphragm. This does not allow the diaphragm to move. The diaphragm allows for breathing when asleep because the brain stem drives the diaphragm while you sleep.

With the diaphragm paralyzed by fat, breathing stops with sleep and the sleeper awakens. This is Ondine's Curse, a paralyzed diaphragm and a life without sleep.

Fat accumulates in the liver resulting in an enlarged and fatty liver. This is called Non-Alcoholic Fatty Liver Disease, NAFLD, and is accompanied by Steatosis, accumulation of fat in the liver, with or without fibrosis, steatohepatitis. The medical literature reports death from liver failure and renal failure due to obesity.

Obesity stresses the kidneys directly due to the direct metabolic stress on the kidneys created by obesity. In addition, obesity increases hypertension and diabetes which also injure the kidneys. Obesity increases chronic kidney disease and death from kidney failure.

Obesity increases coronary heart disease.

Obesity increases death from heart attacks and heart failure.

Obesity increases the risk of stroke and all the complications of stroke including death

Diet, exercise, and weight loss can reverse all the above side effects and risks of obesity.

By-pass surgery for obesity has severe life-threatening side effects and a high failure rate.

Obesity affects the prostate gland and causes both Benign Prostatic Hypertrophy with urinary obstruction and Prostate Cancer according to literature easily found on the internet.

There is no organ in the body that is spared due to the direct effects of fat accumulation and the indirect effects of diabetes and cardiovascular disease,

Medical interventions for obesity are not very effective and as a result a variety of gastric surgeries have emerged as a last resort for obesity. They have serious side effects and a rather high failure rate.

The Gold Standard for obesity is eighty to ninety percent eat less and ten to twenty percent exercise more.

The only effective intervention for obesity is to eat less and be hungry. There is no way to lose weight except to eat less.

There is no way to eat less without being hungry. If you are not losing weight you are not hungry enough and you are eating too much.

No excuses, no explanations, nature cannot be defeated. You cannot lie to nature.

You can lie to your spouse, your children, your employer, your insurance company, and your doctor. You cannot lie to the weight scales.

Either you are losing weight, or you are eating too much,

I have never had a morbidly obese patient with diabetes, hypertension, headaches, impaired vision, a fatty liver, chronic renal disease, with difficulty breathing tell me they were happy.

I have not been successful in treating obesity.

I refer obese patients to eating disorders clinics as I do not have the tools to resolve obesity.

What does the medical literature tell us about the treatment of obesity? Good question,

Obesity is associated with Bing Eating, Bulimia, Anorexia Nervosa and a host of medical problems starting with early onset Diabetes Mellites with all the complications that go with diabetes.

Obesity and anorexia are in the posture that male erectile dysfunction was before the discovery of Viagra. No simple and effective treatment exists.

Obesity and anorexia are poorly understood neurophysiological dysfunctions.

When the neurophysiological dysfunctions are understood there will be a, "Viagra-neurophysiological-obesity pill," and a "Viagra-neurophysiological-anorexia pill," that will resolve obesity and anorexia as efficiently as Viagra resolves male impotence.

Recent review of the medical literature reveals that treatment of obesity is not very effective and the long-term impact of interventions are not known.

"Overview of meta-analysis on prevention and treatment of childhood obesity."
Bahia L1, Schaan CW2, Sparrenberger K3, Abreu GA4, Barufaldi LA5, Coutinho W6, Schaan BD7.
J Pediatr (Rio J). 2019 Jul - Aug;95(4):385-400. doi: 10.1016/j.jped.2018.07.009. Epub 2018 Aug 16.

Most studies on obesity are short term, and there is no single intervention that has been able to prevent surgery.

Surgery for morbid obesity is effective. But not a cure. Effective is a partial and uncertain reduction in weight. Surgery sometimes needs to be repeated and surgical complications are substantial and include death. "The effectiveness and risks of bariatric surgery: an updated systematic review and meta-analysis," 2003-2012. Chang SH1, Stoll CR1, Song J2, Varela JE3, Eagon CJ3, Colditz GA1.
JAMA Surg. 2014 Mar;149(3):275-87. doi: 10.1001/jamasurg.2013.3654.

In summary, you are better off if you control your dietary intake.

Learn to fast in moderation.

Learn to stop eating when you are still hungry to lose weight.

If you are underweight, learn to eat when you are not hungry.

Eat the calories you require to achieve and maintain your ideal weight.

The hardest lessen in life is learning to control your appetites and your impulses.

Master yourself and you master the art of living.

After eating, sleeping is the next life activity with common issues that result in a doctor's appointment.

Most normal people experience insomnia for a day or more depending upon circumstances. Twenty five percent of people have insomnia and three out of four recover, and one out of four suffer an extended period of insomnia.

Chronic insomnia is reported to range from three to thirty three percent of population samples. The patient populations sampled vary as does the definition of insomnia.

Associations that treat insomnia tend to report a higher rate of insomnia than groups that do not treat insomnia.

Babies are born without ninety-minute REM cycles that are the basis of normal sleep in adults.

Babies have fifty-minute REM cycles that mature to ninety-minute REM cycles in their ninth month on average.

Maturation of physiologic functions have a wide range on the calendar.

Physiologic functions are not tied directly to the calendar and are affected by a wide variety of intervening variables including diet, weather, family, DNA, community and cultural environments.

It is believed that REM sleep is a time during which the brain processes the daily experiences into memories and consolidates the daily learning with lifetime experiences.

The details are not completely known. It is known that memories are reconstructed and generally not recalled with digital accuracy.

Memories are generally analogue representations of a single event through the lens of a life of learning.

Insomnia is defined as lack of normal sleep.

Physiologic functions fall on a spectrum of extremes from the rare complete absence to the rare complete presence.

For insomnia there would be the complete absence due to Ondine's curse to the complete presence due to a coma from a head injury.

Ondine's Curse is due to damage anywhere from the respiratory center located in the medulla oblongata to paralysis of the phrenic nerve to the diaphragm.

Ondine's Curse occurs if the person stops breathing when he falls into asleep. When the breathing stops the person wakes up. The result is a life without sleep.

Adults with Guillain Barre post viral polyneuropathy can stop breathing due to damage to this same neurological array from the brain to the diaphragm.

The respiratory arrest wakes the patient up.

It is necessary to put the patient into an iron lung to breathe for the patient or have some other mechanical respiration when he wants to sleep.

Tracheotomy and ventilators have the drawback of infections and other complications.

Iron lungs were used to keep polio patients alive when they couldn't breathe because of damage to the neurological array between the brain and diaphragm.

Sleep apnea from mechanical pressure on the diaphragm from fat in the liver and abdomen can also cause respiratory arrest and insomnia, Pickwickian Syndrome is an early description of respiratory problems from fat in the abdomen paralyzing the diaphragm.

Acid reflux can cause insomnia due to irritation of the vocal cords and respiratory distress.

Restless legs and other movement disorders during sleep can cause insomnia.

Malfunction of the sleep cycle due to neurophysiologic impairments, medical problems, medications, sleep apnea and street drugs can cause insomnia.

Insomnia can be due to an abnormal circadian rhythm that con be shorter than 24 hours, longer than 24 hours or otherwise pathological sleep patterns.

Abnormal behavior patterns can lead to insomnia from mental illness or bad habits.

Shift work and poor sleep hygiene can cause insomnia. Work in foundries, emergency rooms and other environments often require that the employee rotate through the first, second and third shift every ninety days or so. The rotation can be retrograde or anterograde.

If the employee is required to move to a later shift and stay up longer the transition to normal sleep is easier than if the employee is required to go to an earlier shift and start sleeping earlier.

It is easier to sleep later than earlier than the normal bedtime.

This leads to the topic of sleep hygiene.

Sleep hygiene is a pattern of behavior that promotes or disrupts healthy sleep.

For optimum sleep a person should get up and go to bed at the same time every day.

In general, it is best to get up with the sun rise and go to sleep after dark. Eight to ten hours of sleep on average is optimum for good physical and mental health.

The bell-shaped curve for healthy sleep is in fact six to ten hours of sleep for the general population.

Healthy sleep is different for each person. Each person has a normal range of sleep that varies from night to night.

It is necessary to keep a sleep diary to determine what a person's normal sleep is for optimum physical and mental health.

It is necessary to keep a sleep diary to determine what is the normal variation in hours of sleep per night for each individual.

The sleep diary should record the number and time of beverages with caffeine.

The sleep diary should include the time and amount of physical activity and meals.

The sleep diary should include the time and amount of medications taken.

The sleep diary should include the type of work and duration for each day.

The sleep diary should include the types and severity of daily stressors and the types and significance of positive social, educational, vocational, and health events.

The sleep diary should include the duration and quality of sleep and the energy and fatigue levels upon arising, during the day and at bedtime.

There should be daily, weekly, and monthly reviews of the sleep diary.

The activities and experiences that improve sleep or cause insomnia should be tracked during the year and the effects of interventions to improve sleep should also be tracked.

Sleep hygiene generally requires going to sleep and getting up at the same time each morning.

Two or three cups of coffee in the morning has been associated with a reduction of depression and suicide.

Switching from caffeinated beverages in the morning to chamomile tea in the afternoon and evening is associated with improved sleep.

Taking melatonin in the evening is associated with improved sleep.

If sleep hygiene does not maintain healthy sleep, I recommend a sleep EEG and a consultation with a sleep clinic to sort out the different medical conditions and sleep disorders that impair sleep.

You could be suffering from Narcolepsy and a host of other medical problems with specific interventions that improve sleep.

I recommend against the long-term use of a sleeping pill.

Sleeping pills are addicting and lose their effect within fourteen days.

Insomnia is in the posture of male impotence before the discovery of Viagra.

Lacking Viagra for Insomnia, it is necessary to have a sleep EEG and a consultation with a sleep clinic to properly diagnose and treat insomnia.

Zolpidem/Ambien and benzodiazepines are used for insomnia. They are addicting and I do not recommend them for long term use.

Other problems with Zolpidem/Ambien and benzodiazepines include confusion, falls and hip fractures in the elderly. In any age group there are dissociative states reported including sleep eating, sleep sex, sleep driving. Attorneys have used the "Ambien Defense," to acquit defendants from charges of homicide.

More than seventy percent of patients on Ambien continue Ambien after fourteen days although it is known to lose effect after fourteen days. I ask, "physicians prescribe medications, but patients ignore FDA safety recommendations?" What say you?

"77% of patients ignore FDA safety recommendations for Ambien"
Moore TJ, et al. JAMA Intern Med. 2018;doi:10.1001/jamainternmed.2018.3031. July 19, 2018

I say that the literature supporting medication for insomnia is based upon short term studies that cannot address issues of addiction properly. What say you?

"Benzodiazepines and zolpidem for chronic insomnia: a meta-analysis of treatment efficacy."
Nowell PD1, Mazumdar S, Buysse DJ, Dew MA, Reynolds CF 3rd, Kupfer DJ.
JAMA. 1997 Dec 24-31;278(24):2170-7.

Cognitive Behavior Therapy seems to be the most effective treatment for insomnia.

Cognitive and behavioral therapies in the treatment of insomnia: A meta-analysis
Annemieke van Straten, Tanja van der Zweerde a, Annet Kleiboer a, Pim Cuijpers a,

Charles M. Morin b , Jaap Lancee.

Long term use of sleeping pills are generally contraindicated as the adverse effects of addiction and habituation outweigh the benefits which are generally short-term effectiveness that wanes and dissipates with habituation and addiction after the first two weeks.

"Behavioral and pharmacologic therapies for chronic insomnia in adults,"
<u>Michael H Bonnet, PhD</u>
<u>Donna L Arand, PhD</u>
Section Editor:
<u>Ruth Benca, MD, PhD</u>
Deputy Editor:
<u>April F Eichler, MD, MPH</u>

In summary, moderation in all things supports a healthy sleep pattern.

Going to bed and getting up the same time every day is very important for high quality sleep, physical and mental health.

Personal discipline in these matters is part of the lifelong task of mastering yourself. You can do it.

Now we address the topic of exercise.

Daily exercise reduces anxiety, reduces depression, and improves sleep.

Exercise should be started slowly with light exercise and should be increased slowly.

This allows the tendons and ligaments to increase in strength and prevent injuries.

Muscles tend to increase in strength faster than ligaments and tendons.

Aggressive exercise can lead to injuries to tendons and ligaments.

Start with low levels of exercise and increase exercise slowly. This cautious approach to exercise prevents injury and allows for integration of exercise into the daily routine with minimal disruption of other life activities.

One pound, two pound, three pound, four pound, five pound, six pound, seven pound, eight pound, nine pound and ten pound dumbbell sets are inexpensive.

These dumb bells allow for start low and go-slow routines at home. Generally, an exercise routine at home can be done in the time that it takes to travel to the gym.

The exercise routine can be done in the morning before work with a few cups of coffee.

Daily exercise as a lifelong routine is the most effective strategy for moderation and for good physical and mental health.

Exercise is effective for reducing depression and anxiety.

"Effects of exercise on depression and anxiety in persons living with HIV: A meta-analysis," Heissel A1, Zech P2, Rapp MA2, Schuch FB3, Lawrence JB2, Kangas M4, Heinzel S5. J Psychosom Res. 2019 Nov;126:109823. doi: 10.1016/j.jpsychores.2019.109823. Epub 2019 Sep 2.

The literature that describes a small effect for medications on depression and anxiety implies the fact that exercise may be as effective as medications for depression and anxiety.

Analysis of the research concludes that the research is of poor quality and medications are not much more effective than placebo for depression for mild, moderate and severe depression.

"Initial severity of major depression and efficacy of new generation antidepressants: individual participant data meta-analysis." Furukawa TA, Maruo K, Noma H, Tanaka S, Imai H, Shinohara K, Ikeda K, Yamawaki S, Levine SZ, Goldberg Y, Leucht S, Cipriani A. Acta Psychiatr Scand. 2018 Jun;137(6):450-458. doi: 10.1111/acps.12886. Epub 2018 Apr 3.

"Efficacy and Safety of Selective Serotonin Reuptake Inhibitors, Serotonin-Norepinephrine Reuptake Inhibitors, and Placebo for Common Psychiatric Disorders Among Children and Adolescents A Systematic Review and Meta-analysis,"
Cosima Locher, PhD1; Helen Koechlin, MSc; Sean R. Zion, MA; et al Christoph Werner, BSc; Daniel S. Pine, MD; Irving Kirsch, PhD; Ronald C. Kessler, PhD; Joe Kossowsky, PhD, MMSc
JAMA Psychiatry. 2017;74(10):1011-1020. doi:10.1001/jamapsychiatry.2017.2432

If you have medical conditions such as heart conditions, skeletal malformations and other medical conditions you should consult with a cardiologist, orthopedic surgeon or physiatrist for a recommendation regarding exercise and possibly work with a physical therapist to learn how to exercise correctly to avoid physical injury.

In general, swimming is the best exercise because it takes the weight off joints while allowing for a good cardiovascular workout.

In general, aerobic exercise that increases the heart rate is superior to non-aerobic exercise.

Moderation in all things, mastering yourself and daily small changes lead to the optimum life style and best quality of life.

Religion can be seen through the lens of history as science before the scientific method.

Religious clerics in the middle ages brought Greek philosophy and math and science back to life and started the renaissance of science in the western culture.

"The Golden Rule," is a bridge between science and religion. The golden rule is a basic tenet in most religions. "The Golden Rule," is implied in Sun Tzu's book, <u>The Art of War.</u> Sun Tzu stated that war was a failure of politics. This also implied moderation as war is an extreme measure.

"The Golden Rule," is a part of a winning strategy in the science of game theory. Game theory is the science of conflict as manifested in politics, war and sports.

The point of discussing the, "Golden Rule," here is that it is an important part of moderation in all things. Making friends instead of enemies is part of moderation in all things. In general, it is better to give a little more than you receive.

Casting bread upon the waters embraces the idea that it comes back sevenfold.

Charity and hospitality are investments in the community with intangible as well as tangible rewards.

A community with charity and hospitality is a stable, low conflict community that fosters good mental health.

Moderation in all things includes pursuing a variety of interests and activities.

Variety is the spice of life.

Variety is an antidote to boredom.

Zen Buddhism embraces beauty in simplicity. Simplicity allows for low energy meditation and peace of mind that balances the complexity and stimulation created by contests in sports and politics.

A balance of simplicity and complexity, a balance of peace and stress, balance among all dimensions is a means of achieving moderation in all things while exploring boundaries and variety.

Moderation in sleep, eating and exercise all contribute to good health.

Exploring boundaries and your tolerance to boredom and stress as you approach boundaries is part of learning to master your interests, appetites and addictions.

Wisdom and peace of mind can be yours.

Mastery of your interests, appetites and addictions is mastery of life.

Mastery of your interests and addictions is a means of acquiring wisdom and peace of mind as you mature into late life.

Wisdom and peace of mind embrace all that is important in life.

Thank you for your time and attention.

William R. Yee, M.D., J.D.
Board Certified Psychiatrist
Practicing psychiatry without interruption in Michigan, Indiana, Kentucky, California and Texas since 1972, at your service.

I am here to do no harm and help if I can.

"Preexisting text," includes names of symptoms, medical illnesses, medications, people, corporations, law cases, statutes, text of statutes, the titles of articles and books, the content of articles and books cited.

My copyright claim is a clam to the "original text," which is my personal experiences as described in the text above and my commentary on the preexisting text listed above.

www.ingramcontent.com/pod-product-compliance
Lightning Source LLC
Chambersburg PA
CBHW070431180526
45158CB00017B/974